THE MYSTIC ART OF PULSE READING IN CHINA

BY

L.C. ARLINGTON

Edited by

Mark Linden O'Meara

Foreword by Ioannis Solos Phd

Original published in

THE CHINA JOURNAL OF SCIENCE & ARTS
VOL. II, No. 5 (September, 1924), pp. 400-411

Soul Care Publishing
Vancouver, Canada
SoulCarePublishing.com

Table of Contents

Foreword

Lewis Charles Arlington, (author of In Search of Old Peking) is an American who worked in Beijing at the end of the Qing and the beginning of the Republic of China. In this essay he attempted to introduce the subject of Chinese pulses to a western audience. Strictly judging from the medical content of his work, his recitation of the various Chinese pulses is commendable as a quick summary of the basic information on the subject. Although it is not a comprehensive study of pulses that could be used to guide clinical treatment, it provides a glimpse into the vast and complex subject through western eyes.

This version of his article had been skillfully edited to remove Arlington's obvious biases against Chinese medicine and the Chinese culture. By doing so we are left with a text that conveys a basic understanding of pulses that allows the lay person to gain an understanding of this complex field of Traditional Chinese Medicine.

Arlington wrote his original text at a time when doctors in the west still believed that syphilis was due to the degeneration of the thyroid gland and not -as we know today- a *Treponema pallidum* infection. The author's overconfidence in the superiority of his erroneous beliefs over the Chinese theories is a timely reminder that in science there are no absolutes. With Chinese medicine becoming massively popular worldwide and with the advancements of conventional medicine, some of the author's rudest comments are now quite embarrassing and fortunately are removed from this edition.

In regards to the 21st century, it's very disconcerting that Arlington's terms such as "quackery" used in the text to describe Chinese medicine could also very well portray many of the early 20th century western practices. It's also very disturbing that the same term still persists in current literature although clinical evidence to the contrary has become abundant.

The editing and publication of this text by Mark Linden O'Meara comes at a time when it's important to look back and re-examine the relentless criticism that Chinese medicine had to face even before Nixon's historic trip to China, and also ascertain that modern arguments are often no better than Arlington's imperialist attempts to vilification.

Ioannis Solos Phd
Doctor of Medicine, Chinese Medical Author, Sinologist
Guangzhou, China 26/10/2018

Introduction

The exact date when the feeling of the pulse to test the circulation of the blood through the arteries originated in China is unknown. It is, however, recorded in the Lieh Kuo Chih that a man named Chin Yuen-jen who lived in the 5th century B.C., received from an old man named Ch'ang Shang-chun a certain drug which he was instructed to take for thirty consecutive days, and, on the expiry of which he was able to understand the "Nature of Things." The old man also presented him with books on medicine, and the art of healing, with which he set forth and travelled from State to State as a doctor, performing all kinds of wonderful cures. He is commonly known to the Chinese by his pseudonym Pien Ch'ueh.

He is said to have been able to look into the viscera of his patients, and the knowledge of the pulse is inseparably associated with his name. He was assassinated at the instigation of Li Hsi, Chief Physician at the Court of Ch'in, out of jealousy of his unrivalled skill. We find it recorded in the Lieh Kuo Chih, above mentioned, that Chin Ching Kung, the grandson of Chin Wen Kung, one of the Five famous rulers in the 7th century B.C., whose real name was Chung Erh (See B. D, No. 523), during a spell of sickness dreamt that two page-boys, the embodiment of his disease, hid in his vitals in such places as to be beyond the reach of either drugs or acupuncture; hence, the saying "Twin calamity"

3

means an incurable disease. He further dreamt that the twins came out of his nostrils and at once began the following conversation: "A famous doctor is coming to diagnose our father's illness," said one, "which will be very serious for us." "Well" said the other, "I'll tell you what we'll do, let one of us hide above the heart, and the other below it." Hence, the saying "When the disease has entered the vitals it is a sure sign of death." Now it happened that two of Pien Ch'ueh's medical students Kao Ho and Kao Huan arrived to diagnose the case, The latter on feeling the sick man's pulse at once remarked "the disease has entered your vitals, nothing can save you, your hour is at hand." "That's wonderful," said the patient, "what you say exactly corresponds with my dream!" That same night he expired.

Chinese medical authors have been numerous from very remote periods, and there seems little doubt that the art had been reduced to some sort of system before the days of Solomon. It is even recorded that the Emperor Shen Nung (2838 B.C.) wrote a treatise on Medicine. They have volumes describing minutely the practice of amputation and the nature of internal diseases said to have been written by Huang Ti (2698 B.C.). They have also several works on diseases of the Eye: several on Fevers; scores of volumes on the diseases of women; many volumes on diseases of the skin; on diseases of the blood vessels; nervous diseases; diseases of the mouth, teeth and the throat; the treatment of fractures and wounds. In addition to the famous Materia Medica entitled "Pen Ts'ao Kang Mu" written in the middle of the I6th century in 52 hooks, there is a celebrated work on Therapeutics called "Pu Tse-fang" said to have been written by the Ming Prince Chu Su. It consists of 160 volumes and contains about 1,800 lectures on some 2,000 subjects; 21,000 different prescriptions; 775 rules, and 235 diagrams. During the late Manchu dynasty the faculty of medicine was fixed by the Government to consist of 9 branches, namely: diseases of the skin; diseases of the large blood vessels; diseases of the small blood vessels; diseases of the eye; diseases of the mouth, teeth and throat; diseases of the bones; diseases of women; fever and cases for acupuncture. There is also a work of 20 books on Hygiene, which treats of diet, rest, study, proper clothing, amusements, how to prevent disease, etc. It was published in 1591.

There are also works on smallpox illustrated with diagrams of the disease, and prescriptions for its treatment, as well as works on cholera discussing methods of treating the disease, several volumes on the diseases of partutrition giving directions for the management of children. Other works on Medical art might be mentioned, but enough has been said to show that there is no lack of quantity. Chinese physicians say that Man's body is composed of the Five Viscera, which partake of the nature of the Five Elements, i.e., fire, water, metal, wood and earth, and these they connect with the Five Tastes, Five Colors and the Seven Passions {see infra): diseases they say are produced by a derangement m the balancing of all these elements. Certain mysterious dual powers in nature called the Yin and Yang, corresponding to light and darkness, earth and heaven, male and female, strength and weakness, etc., also play an important part both in medicine and pulse feeling.

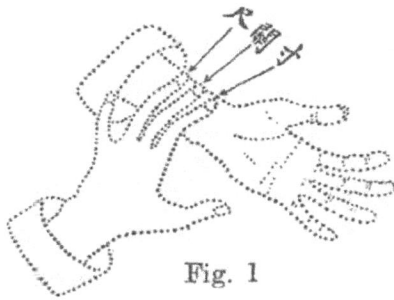 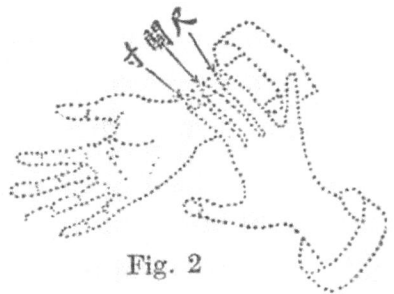

Fig. 1   Fig. 2

The heart is the prince of the body and the seat of learning. The soul is supposed to reside in the liver; the gal. is the seat of courage; the seat of life is in the stomach.

But of all the systems none is so evident or prevalent both in theory and practice as their doctrine of the pulse; and, as stated at the head of this paper, it is the pulse we are concerned. They claim that there is a different and distinct pulse for every part of the body which is felt on both wrists, believing that not only does the pulse differ on both wrists or sides; but actually distinguish three on each arm, the first immediately on the metacarpus, and called respectively the "inch" the "bar" and the "cubit" (See Figures 1 and 2).

Chinese physicians assert that the entire superstructure of medical, practice depends on this theory of the pulse, —the diagnosis, prognosis, and treatment of every disease rest entirely on this.

L.C. Arlington

The Chinese Theory of the Pulse

Extent, one inch or three fingers placed side by on the left and right wrists (See Figures 1 and 2).

Division into three parts,—1st called ts'un (inch), 2nd, Kuan (bar or pass), 3rd, ch'ih (cubit).

There are Four Principal Pulses: Ssu Ta Kang viz.: Fu (1) a light flowing (superficial) pulse like something lightly floating on water (2) Ch'en, a deeply impressed pulse like a stone thrown into water (3) Ch'ih, a slow pulse (three beats to one cycle of respiration); and (4) So or Sho, a quick pulse (6 beats to one cycle of respiration).

The 1st, Fu, indicates external (unimportant) complaints, such as colds, etc. The 2nd, Ch'en, indicates internal (serious) complaints; contracted in the Five Viscera, and connected with the seven Passions (see infra), internal injuries, non-mixing of food, drink, etc. The 3rd, Ch'ih, indicates chills. The 4th, Sho, indicates heat.

The diseases contracted through external influences or six influences, Yin and Fang, wind, rain, light, and darkness), are: diseases contracted through dampness, etc.; diseases occurring through the sun's rays, etc.; colds contracted through wind, etc.; chills contracted internally; diseases contracted by being parched by the sun; and complaints arising through too much internal heat, etc. Diseases contracted through internal influences, i.e., the "Seven Passions," are: joy; anger; anxiety; melancholy thoughts; grief; suppressed fear; and being suddenly frightened or startled.

(Note.—According to Chinese ideas Heaven has Six Influences, viz.: sunshine, moon-shine, wind, rain, darkness and light, while human beings have Seven Passions, viz: joy, anger, grief, pleasure, love, hatred and ambition.

The following are the pulse tests for internal and external heat and chills: if the pulse is Fu - superficial, and Sho, quick (6 beats), it indicates external heat; but if it is Ch'en, deep , and Sho, quick, there is internal heat. If it is Fu and Ch'ih (3 beats), there is external chill; but if Ch'en, deep and Ch'ih, there is internal chill. If the left ts'un is Fu and Sho there is disturbance in the region of the heart, such as caused by external heat, If the right ts'un is Fu, superficial, and Sho, quick, it indicates diseases caused by external heat in the chest and lungs; if the Kuan on the left wrist is Ch'en, deep, and Sho, quick, there is internal heat in the liver and gall; but if the Kuan on the right side is Fu and Sho, there is internal heat in the spleen and stomach. If the left ch'ih-Cubit is Fu, superficial, and Ch'ih, slow, it indicates external cold in the kidneys and bladder, If the right ch'ih-Cubit it is Fu and Ch'ih, it indicates external chill in the kidneys and colon.

L.C. Arlington

Pulses of the Four Seasons; Five Elements; and Five Colors.

In the spring when the element wood is predominant, the pulse of the liver is hsien, tremulous motion like a taut fiddle string; the color element being blue. In summer, the element fire is predominant, the pulse of the heart which answers to hung, "overflowing"; the color element being red. In autumn, the element metal is predominant, the pulse of the lungs being mao, "elastic"; the color element being white. In winter, the element water prevails, the pulse of the kidneys which, answers to shih "heavy"; like a stone thrown into the water; the color element being black.

The stomach, however, is governed by the Four Seasons, as that particular organ may be disordered at any time, hence, it answers to t'u, earth, and. the color element being yellow (corresponding to earth); the pulse being Ho Huan, "Slow" and in harmony with Nature.

In addition to the above we have twelve subsidiary pulses to consider; viz., Hung, an overflowing pulse; Hsu, a slow, weak and scattered pulse; Ju, superficial hollow pulse like an onion-stalk, and small in compass; Ko, hollow like an onion-stalk but taut like a fiddle string; Fu, very deep and quick; Lao, deep and strong; Jo, deep and feeble; Se, moderately slow with strength; Chin, quick with strength; Ts'u, hasty, the pulse beat

10

irregular, with indications of strength, hsien, taut and tremulous like a. musical string; and finally, hua, slippery, like a pebble rolling around in a basin with irregular movements. "Care" the books say, "must be taken not to confuse the different kinds of pulse which resemble each other." What fickled fancies of a distempered brain!

The kidneys are said to be the seat of energy; therefore, the "bar" on the left wrist is felt; if there is no pulse there is no hope of cure! The Wu T'sang or Five Viscera, which constitute the hsin, heart; kan, liver; p'i, stomach; fei, lungs; and shen, kidneys, play an important part also in pulse feeling, In order to test whether all of the above mentioned are in good condition, the left ts'un is felt for the heart, in which, if healthy, the pulse should be superficial and wide-spreading in compass. The ts'un on the right wrist is felt for the lungs, and should be—if in health—superficial, moderately slow and short; i.e. jerky.

As already stated above, the condition of the liver is tested on the left kuan or "bar" which, if in health, should be deep, and taut like a tremulous musical string, and covering the full width of the finger placed on the pulse. The kidneys are tested on the ch'ih-cubit, of both wrists; and as the kidneys belong to the element water, if in health, the pulse should be deep, superficial, hollow like an 'onion-stalk' and small in compass, i.e., not

11

exceeding the boundaries of the ch'ih-cubit. The condition of the stomach is tested by the "bar" on the right wrist; in health, the pulse should be moderately slow (huan). The pulse on the left Ts'un is tested for complaints of the heart. The same test is made for hsiang huo, the sexual spark or emotion (i.e., whether sexual excesses have been committed). They make confusion worse confounded, they claim that the Ts'un corresponds to Yang, the male principal of nature. The kuan to half of Yang and half of Yin; i.e., half male and half female nature; and that ch'ih-cubit corresponds to Yin, Female Nature.

In former times, and indeed, up till quite recently (1924), men were tested on the left wrist, and women on the right one. This silly practice has now become obsolete, both men and women undergoing the same tests on either wrists, and this in spite of the Male and Female Principals of Nature- what a concession on the part of Chinese physicians!

One authority says that the pulse of a patient should be felt early in the morning, at sunrise. That the doctor should keep cool and collected and show no signs of anxiety (this latter is one of the most, if not the most, sensible remarks to be found in the whole history of Chinese medical art). The doctor should pay particular attention to the patient's breathing, which should be regular, from 4 to 4 and a 1/2 beats to each cycle of respiration; hence, normal. Let us, however, delve a little deeper into this wonderful and mysterious circulation of the blood as discovered by Chinese physicians; A slight catarrh of the lungs is shown by the Fu or superficial pulse. If the right Ts'un is quick, and at the same time strong it indicates a slight cold in the lungs; but if the same pulse is Sho and weak, it shows that the patient is suffering from asthma. (see note 1)

Note 1: Dr. Hobson in an excellent paper in the Medical Times and Gazette in November 1860 says :- "the Chinese have no name for inflammation, and I had to transfer the term, or a contraction of it, before I could describe its symptoms and treatment. They have a term which means hot; but a hot disease is not inflammation, nor have the well-known characteristics of the disease ever been describe in any book that I have seen or heard of in China; so that though they have a large nosological list, this most important pathological affection is not even so much as named."

But to illustrate further: If the right ts'un is Fu but Chin (6 beats with strength), there is catarrh in the lungs and diaphragm, If the same pulse is moderately slow and weak, it indicates rheumatism. If the right Ts'un is superficial, and hollow like an onion-stalk, there is loss of blood; and if the same pulse is Hsu, very weak, it indicates illness brought on through sunstroke. Insufficient blood is indicated by the ts'un pulse if Fu,

L.C. Arlington

superficial and feeble. If either of the ts'un pulses are superficial, and hollow like an onion-stalk, and small in compass, there is insufficiency in both the blood and breath. In the case of colds, when the pulse is Fu, superficial, and Hung, overflowing, there is no danger because it is influenced by Yang, the Male Principal, If the pulse is Ch'en, deep, and thin and thready, it shows that the cold has entered the vitals, and is difficult to cure, In eases of apoplexy, if the pulse is Fu, superficial and slow, Ch'ih, 3 beats, no danger exists; but if it is very deep, hasty and large in compass, there is little hope left. In cases of fever, the signs are favourable if the pulse is hsein, taut like a tremulous musical string, and at the same time is Sho, 6 beats; if the same pulse is Ch'ih, slow, 3 beats, it indicates an attack of malaria. It is very serious, however, if the pulse stops and beats at regular periods, barely perceptible and scattered (less than three beats).

If in cases of diarrhea, any of the pulses are Ch'en, deep but small in compass, or Jo, irregular and weak, the disease is curable; but if it is Fu and Sho, superficial and quick, there is great danger, more especially if the patient cannot eat any food, In eases of vomiting, there is no danger if the pulse is Fu and hua, superficial and rolling about like a slippery pebble in a dish. If the pulse is hsien and Sho, taut like a tremulous musical string and quick (6 beats); or Chin Se, i.e., very irregular sometimes with

14

strength, or sometimes slow or moderately slow with strength, it indicates that there is no blood left in the intestines. Whether an attack of cholera is serious or not, is determined as follows: if the pulse is overflowing and large in compass, the attack is slight; hut if the pulse is slow -and feeble; the cure is difficult. Where there is a severe cough, if the pulse is Fu, Ju, superficial and hollow, also weak, there is no danger; but if the pulse is Ch'en, Se, deep with much strength, there is danger of running into consumption. Where asthma exists, if the pulse is Fu, hua superficial and slippery, like a stone rolling about in a basin, no danger is apprehended; but if it is Ch'en, Se, deep, sharp, and slow with strength, and if the hands and feet are cold at the same time, there is great danger of death. If the body is overheated, should the pulse be Hung, Sho, overflowing and quick, there is nothing to fear; but, if very small and feeble, a cure is difficult.

In wasting diseases, especially of the lungs if the pulse is superficial and very weak, the disease is easily cured; but if Hung, Sho, floating and quick, there may be serious complications.

In eases of loss of blood; if the pulse is hollow like an onion-stalk and moderately slow and small in compass; no further loss may occur; but if hollow, and quick, also large in compass, more blood will be lost, hence, dangerous. Congestion of the blood in the region of the heart: if the pulse is, deep and strong and large in compass, a cure may be expected, but if deep very slow, and irregular, there is great danger to the patient. In cases of stoppage of the urine, Bright's disease, etc: if the pulse is quick (6 beats), and large in compass, the disease is curable, but if fine and small, the case is almost hopeless. In cases of venereal diseases, if the pulse is very tight, strong and large in compass the disease is easily cured; but if very slow, irregular, and small in compass, a cure is difficult.

The Chinese physicians apparently do not know that syphilis, with which many Chinese are infected, is also due to the degeneration of the thyroid gland. In cases of insanity, if the pulse is Fu, Hung, superficial and overflowing, a cure may be expected, but if the pulse is Ch'en, deep and hasty, the case is hopeless. Here, again, the Chinese doctors are at sea; they can probably note that there is a disturbance in the blood circulation of the brain-cortex, due to changes in the blood vessels, but it is very doubtful if they can note the destruction of the nerve-cells and nerve processes. Nor do they know that the degeneration of the thyroid is the fundamental cause of this disease. Convulsions, spasms, fits, etc: if the pulse is superficial, slow, and large in compass, there is no danger, but if deep and small in compass, or taut like a tremulous musical string and hasty, or quick, there is great danger, especially if the liver is disordered. In cases of rupture in the groin, hernia, etc: if the pulse is overflowing and hasty, a cure is possible, but if weak and hasty, death is near! In eases of swellings, such as a dropsical belly: if the pulse is superficial and large in compass, also overflowing and strong or tight, no great danger exists, but if Ch'en, deep, and fine and thready, danger exists.

In cases of jaundice: if the pulse is superficial and large in compass, or Sho, hung quick and overflowing, the diseases may be cured, but if the pulse is sharp, irregular and small in compass, there is danger of death.

Accumulation of humours in the body: so long as any of the Six Pulses show strong pulsations, there is no danger, but if any one of them is Ch'en, deep, and fine and thready, the case is serious. Disorders derived through evil-influences, such as ghosts, demons, etc. are said to be serious if the pulse is Fu, superficial and large in compass, or Fu, hung, superficial and overflowing. But if the pulse is Chin, quick, strong, and flue, there is no danger.

Cancer, carbuncle, etc: if the pulse is Hung, overflowing and large in compass, the case is not considered, dangerous, but if blood or pus exudes (with the same pulse) it is critical.

In cases of abscess on the lungs: if the ts'un pulse on the right- side is short, slow, and irregular, but small in compass, i.e, not overflowing the space included in the ts'un there are hopes of a cure, but if the same pulse is Fu, superficial and large in compass, the patient may as well prepare for death! Cancer in the stomach: if the left ts'un or right Cubit is Sho, quick, and hua, slippery, no danger may be apprehended, but if the same pulses are Ch'en, deep and fine there is little hope of recovery.

The Four Essential Points The Physician Must Pay Regard To

1st: to note the expression of the face, complexion, condition of the tongue, etc, 2nd: to note if there are any bad smells corning from the nose, mouth, body, or in the house the patient is living in, 3rd: to make inquiries into the probable cause of the illness, when the symptoms first manifested, in which part of the body, and whether the patient is fond of hot food and drinks, 4th: to diagnose the case by the above-mentioned three tests, combined with the actions of the various pulses, and prescribe the remedy. In cases of stoppage of menstruation, if the three pulses on both wrists, Ts'un, Kuan, and Cubit, are slippery like a pebble rolling about in a basin and quick (6 beats), it shows three months conception. If the three pulses, as indicated above, are highly pulsating it indicates 5 months conception. If the pulses on the left wrist are exceedingly quick, a male child may be expected, but if the right pulses are exceedingly rapid a female child in ay be looked for. (See Note 2)

Note 2: The Chinese believe that if a woman during pregnancy is suddenly called from a. sitting or reclining position, and upon arising unconsciously puts her left foot out first, she is with a male child, and if it should be the right foot, it will be a girl. They also have a saying to the effect that it is much better to rear a male child after 280 days have elapsed than a daughter under the belief that the former is lucky, but not the latter. This is because they reckon the period for conception to birth at 9 months of 30 days each, plus ten days, or a total of 280 days.

If the pulses on both wrists mingle or run together (i.e., the ts'un pulse coalesces with the Kuan or the latter with the Cubit or vice versa), it indicates 9 months pregnancy, and birth may be expected within ten days. After the birth of a child, if the mother's Six Pulses are small in compass, and moderately slow, she is safe, but if the Six Pulses are firm, large in compass, and taut like a tremulous musical string, she is in a very critical condition.

Indications of Pulse: If the pulse is weak, the "touch" must be very light; the pulse should be drifting and buoyant, like wood floating on the water or like elm-seeds floating on water. A distinction is also made between a pulse that is not exactly Fu, superficial, yet resembles it! If the pulse is Fu with some strength, or overflowing, with 3 beats (Ch'ih), it indicates weakness in the entire system. If the pulse is very much scattered, there is not sufficient oil in the system to lubricate it. If the pulse is hollow like an onion-stalk, and superficial, Fu, the pulsation, barely perceptible on the tip of the finger, and covering a space no larger than a small pea, it indicates extreme weakness in the entire bodily economy, but these pulsations are difficult to distinguish.

If the pulse is "hollow" and taut like a tremulous musical string, the loss of blood has been excessive. If the hollow feel is superficial, in other words, ho mo, pulse in harmony, there is no great danger, but if the 'hollow' feel is Ch'en, deep, with lao, force, there is absolutely no hope of recovery.

If the pulse indications are very deep, like a stone cast into the water, the pressure of the fingers must also be heavy and deep, the pulse can then be felt. If the pulse beats are irregular, stop and then beat again, it indicates, in a woman, that she is *enceinte (childbearing)*, and, in a man, serious injury in the vitals.

The blood is controlled by yin, cold, and the breath by yang, heat. The pulse in actual sickness is as follows: if the pulse is Fu, superficial, it indicates disease of the lungs externally contracted. If the Fu pulse is strong it indicates that a cold has been caught through wind, cold air, etc. If the Fu pulse is very weak, there is deficiency of the blood corpuscles. If the Fu, superficial pulse is Ch'ih, slow (3 beats), cold has been contracted externally, If the same pulse is Sho, quick (6 beats), it indicates internal heat caused by cold air through the pores of the skin. If the Fu pulse is Chin, quick with strength, it indicates an external cold; if the Fu pulse is moderately slow, it indicates rheumatism. If the Fu pulse is superficial and slow, and large in compass, it denotes illness brought on through the sun, such as heat apoplexy. If the Fu is hollow like an onion-stalk, much blood has been lost. If the Fu is Hung, overflowing, it denotes weakness and internal heat caused by sexual excesses. If the Fu is small and feeble, there is loss of vitality through over-work, mental or physical. If the Fu pulse is Ju, hollow like an onion-stalk, and small in compass, there is insufficiency of semen.

Pulses Which Indicate Danger of Death

If the left Kuan is sharp as a knife, it indicates serious complications in the liver, and death may be expected within eight days. If all the Six Pulses or the right kuan in particular, resembles the noise of a bird pecking, the noise of running waters, or is like the sound of water dripping from a roof, or like the noise of the upsetting of a cup containing water, it indicates serious congestion in the bowels, and death may he expected within seven days. If the Six Pulses, or the right ts'un especially, resemble hairs blown by the wind there is congestion of the lungs and the stomach, and death comes within three days. If both the right and left Cubit resemble the sudden snapping of a cord, or like the flipping of the finger against a stone, there is non-action of the kidneys, and death may be predicted within four days. If the Six Pulses act like a fish or shrimp darting about in the water, or like water bursting forth from a spring, death is certain within one or two days. Who can say, with this theory before them, that the Chinese physicians know anything about the true circulation of the blood. If, in addition to the pulse indications, the perspiration is of an oily nature, the eyes are dim, there is a sweetish taste in the mouth, a numbness of the tongue, and the breath is cold, it shows the patient to be in extremes! Ex pede Herculem! (Publisher's note: Ex pede Herculem – "from his foot, we can measure

L.C. Arlington

Hercules" is a maxim of proportionality inspired by an experiment attributed to Pythagoras.)

In Spring, they say the lung pulse is mortal, because the pulse of the heart is set aside, for the latter is the son of the liver, which has the kidneys for its mother, and the stomach for its wife. Then, again, they say if you wish to know whether a patient will recover, you must carefully examine the various actions of the pulse. If the pulse frisks about like a fish that dives, and comes up very slowly, so slow in fact, that one would think it was held back by the tail, and yet makes its escape, such a pulse is absolutely useless, since the most skillful doctor "under the Heavens" could not save the patient. Too many beatings of the pulse proceeds from excess of heat, and too few from excess of cold. This is a constant tradition handed down from all ages, the various degrees of which are set down clearly in the book of the eighty-one difficulties.

Before concluding this paper, I must not omit to mention the following opinion of Dr. Hobson, who practised for 18 years amongst the Chinese: "While they—the Chinese—write learnedly about the wonderful properties of the pulse, and palm a lie upon the public in professing to distinguish its minute and varied forms, yet I have never met with one Chinese medical practitioner who dared affirm to my face that he had done so; or was willing to try his boasted skill on a patient of mine, though offered a considerable reward to point out any well-known. disease by the pulse alone.

It is only fair, however, to see what Chinese physicians think of Western medical art. They believe that our ideas of the true circulation of the blood are based on a "false hypothesis, because they contradict the doctrine of their ancient sages." They ask "How could any post-mortem examination show the blood freely flowing through the veins of a corpse, or ascertain the age of the uterine formation? And scout as ridiculous, the idea that the moral qualities of courage have no dependence on the size of the gall-bladder."

The Chinese, as we know, procure the gall-bladder of such, animals as tigers, bears and snakes, also of men, especially notorious criminals executed for their crimes, to eat the bile contained in them in the belief that it will impart courage.

In conclusion, I beg my readers to pardon my efforts to explain what is unknown by what is even less known.—*Ignotum per ignotius*. (Latin for 'the unknown by the more unknown'.)

www.ingramcontent.com/pod-product-compliance
Lightning Source LLC
Chambersburg PA
CBHW071036050426
42335CB00050B/1794